ROSE REY

The Birth Within

TOP 10 Easy Ways for Expectant Mothers to Craft A Path to Making A Good Human through Motherhood

"You never understand life until it grows inside of you"

SANDRA CHAMI KASSIS (LEBANESE AUTHOR)

Contents

1

Introduction

Welcome to the extraordinary journey that unfolds within the pages of "The Birth Within." In these pages, you will not find just a book; you will discover a sanctuary of shared experiences, a celebration of the universal tapestry of motherhood. "The Birth Within" is a guide and a heartfelt conversation, inviting you into the intimate corridors of pregnancy, parenthood, and the myriad emotions accompanying the miraculous path to becoming a mom.

As the author of this journey, I intend to weave a narrative that resonates with the diverse stories of women worldwide. Each word is a step into the labyrinth of emotions, preparations, and reflections defining the extraordinary motherhood transition.

Throughout this book, you will encounter not only practical advice but also the warmth of shared wisdom, the courage of personal narratives, and the unwavering belief in the beauty of the journey. Here is a space where you, regardless of background or circumstance, can find solace, inspiration, and a sense of connection with the universal experience of motherhood.

As you turn these pages, may you discover not just guidance but a companion for the challenges and joys ahead. "The Birth Within" is an offering, a reflection, and an embrace welcoming you into a community that understands the profound magic of creating life.

So, with an open heart and a spirit of anticipation, let us embark on this shared voyage in the cherished role of mom. May these words resonate with you, inspire you, and accompany you on your unique and beautiful journey into motherhood.

In the future, this book will become a memory bundle of the efforts you made during pregnancy.

Warm regards,
  Rose Rey.

2

The Birth of Genius: How Maternal Care Shapes Destiny

"There is a secret behind the existence of every wonderful, divine, and amazing personality born in the world."

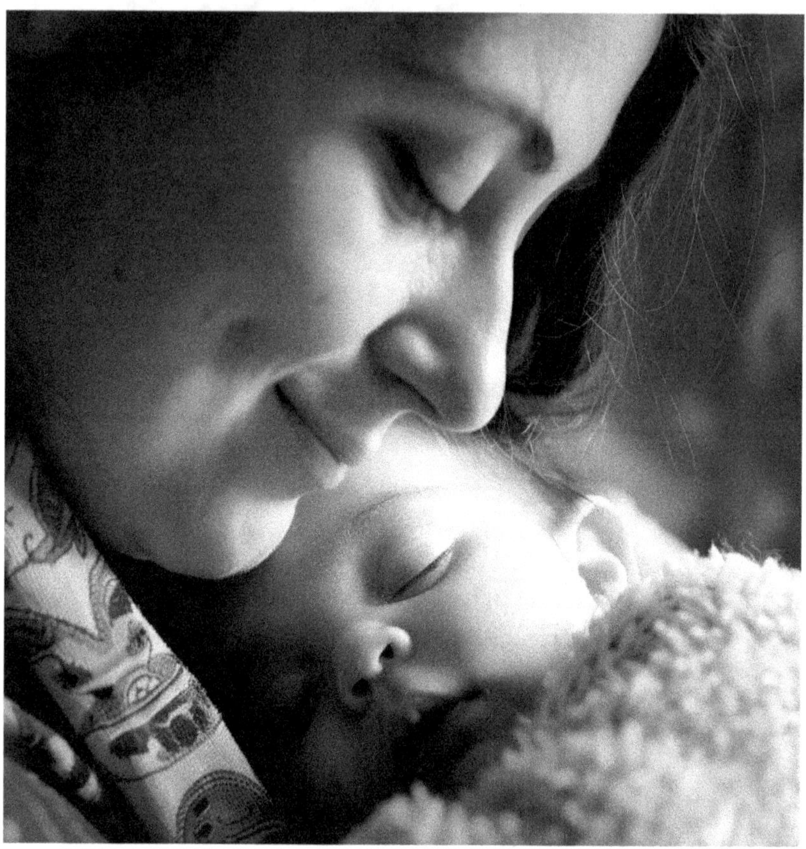

Have you ever noticed some children seem clever and innovative by birth while others need clarification and more confidence?

Let's understand this first with some scientific research.

During pregnancy, stress from things like changes in your personal life, work, or living situation can affect both you and your baby. Research shows that stress, even if it's not severe, can impact your baby's development and your pregnancy. It's important to find ways to manage and cope with stress to help ensure a healthy pregnancy for you and your baby.

Let's understand with an example.

Think of it like planting two beautiful flowers in your garden. One is if it grows in less fertile land, with less sunlight, surrounded by grass. The second one grows your extra care, like fertile land, into the sunlight, required fertilizer, and timely given water.

What do you think? Which plant grows better? It's a second one. We all know that nature plays its role perfectly, and there is no doubt about it. But nowadays, more is needed because of our stressful routine, unhealthy food, and polluted atmosphere. We have to take extra care of our children from the womb.

Providing care is essential for their remarkable development when a child is in the mother's womb. Just as you would give water and proper sunlight to help a planted flower grow similarly, you have to create a healthy atmosphere for your child from the womb.

Finally, this chapter teaches that a child born with extra care is more clever and mentally more potent than a child born with just a system.

Having children is a gift from God, but it requires full effort from its mother.

If you are genuinely prepared to do anything for your child, this book will guide you on how to achieve that. A beautiful science is working on it. You will explore all parts step by step in the following lessons.

Get ready for a fantastic journey full of exciting discoveries and life-changing transformations.

∞∞∞§∞∞∞

3

Building a Solid Foundation

"**M**otherhood is the foundation upon which the future is built."

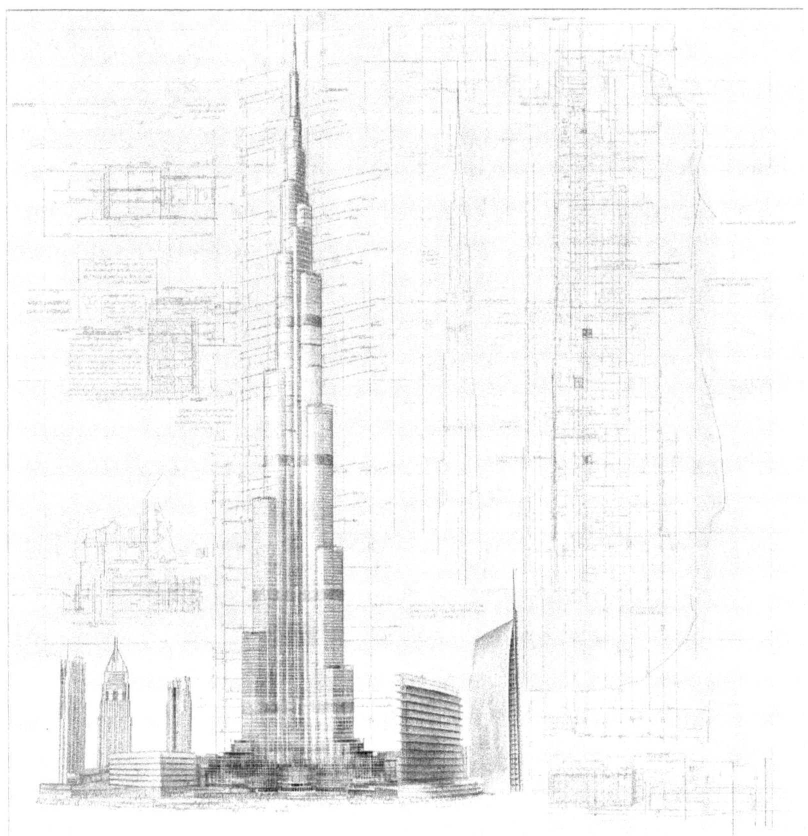

Imagine this,

You spend two decades studying to land a job that might pay 20 to 25 dollars. You work hard to become experts in your fields. Now, think about how much time we invest in preparing for the job of a lifetime, being a parent. No degrees, no official qualifications.

So, let's ask ourselves, have we taken the time to get ready for the incredible responsibility of being a parent, starting with the basics like understanding the role of sex in bringing a baby into the world? As we go through life, have we thought about what it means to be ready for the fantastic journey of caring for a new life?

Building a solid foundation is a bit like constructing a strong and stable house for your family. In the context of preparing for parenthood, it means establishing a reliable base for the journey ahead.

Think of it as laying down the groundwork. Just like a house needs a strong foundation to withstand challenges like weather and time, building a solid foundation in preparation for parenthood involves understanding your values and beliefs about parenting. It's about creating a stable platform that can support you through the ups and downs of raising a child.

Consider this analogy

You're setting up the foundation of a bridge. A sturdy foundation ensures the bridge is strong enough to carry the weight of your family's experiences. Building a solid foundation is similar – it's about reinforcing your relationship, establishing shared values, and creating a reliable base for your parenting journey.

So, building a solid foundation is like constructing a resilient home for your growing family, ensuring that it stands strong amidst the winds of change and provides a secure and nurturing environment for your child.

Let's understand with a story.

A couple named Mia and Gabriel lived in a bustling city where dreams danced in the air. They were about to embark on the extraordinary journey of parenthood. Amidst the excitement, they understood the importance of laying a solid foundation for the family they were about to create.

Mia and Gabriel were inspired by the idea that a strong foundation could weather any storm. They believed that just as a well-built house stands tall against the winds, a family with a solid foundation could thrive through the challenges of parenthood.

They began their journey by defining the core values shaping their family. Communication, respect, and unwavering support were the cornerstones. Mia and Gabriel would spend evenings discussing their dreams for the family, setting intentions to serve as the guiding principles for their parenting adventure.

With these values in mind, Mia and Gabriel sought wisdom from experienced parents in their community. They listened to stories of joy, resilience, and the importance of creating a nurturing environment. These narratives became bricks in their building, a foundation that would withstand the tests of time.

Mia, an artist at heart, envisioned their home as a canvas where memories would be painted with love and laughter. Gabriel, a practical thinker, planned meticulously for financial stability to provide a secure base for their family's future. Together, they realized that building a solid foundation wasn't just about physical structures and weaving a tapestry of emotional security.

They attended parenting workshops, read books on positive discipline, and learned the art of balancing boundaries with love. Each piece of knowledge they gained became another layer in the foundation they were crafting.

Mia's belly grew with the promise of new life, so they transformed a room into a cozy nursery. Gabriel painted the walls with warm colors, while Mia filled the shelves with books that would fuel their child's imagination. This room became a physical representation of the solid foundation they were laying—a space where love and learning would flourish.

When their little one arrived, Mia and Gabriel were greeted with the sweet melody of baby giggles and the scent of newborn innocence. The foundation they had built allowed them to navigate the sleepless nights and the unexpected challenges of parenthood with grace and resilience.

In the following years, their home echoed with the patter of tiny feet and the chatter of growing minds. Mia and Gabriel watched their child take those first steps with the assurance that their foundation would support every stumble and cheer every success.

Mia and Gabriel's commitment to building a solid foundation became even more profound as their family grew. They taught their child the values of kindness, empathy, and the importance of strong connections. Family traditions and shared experiences became the mortar that bound their foundation together.

Years passed, and Mia and Gabriel found themselves surrounded by a family that thrived on the strength of the foundation they had built. The laughter that echoed through their home was a testament to the joy that emanated from a loving and supportive family.

And so, in the heart of the bustling city, Mia, Gabriel, and their child lived a life inspired by the power of building a solid foundation. This story echoed a family's resilience grounded in love, values, and the unwavering belief that they could create a home that stood the test of time with a strong foundation.

Let's do an activity with A Beautiful Smile…

Take a pen & paper, and sit together. Make a checklist about your thoughts, the planning you have done for your baby, financial planning during pregnancy, and the mindset you are in right now.

Are you still trying to think about it? So what are you waiting for?

You may need more guidance. Then, Let's guide you more about how to complete today's Activity.

Visualization Exercise

Close your eyes and take a few deep breaths to center yourself. Imagine your ideal future with your baby.

What does it look like? What values do you hope to instill in them? Picture yourself as the parent you aspire to be, providing love, guidance, and support. Now, jot down your thoughts and feelings about this vision. What steps can you take to manifest this reality? Use this exercise to clarify your goals and intentions, laying the groundwork for a solid foundation for your family.

This Activity focuses on visualization and goal-setting, which can be powerful tools for building a solid foundation for parenthood. Seize the moment your first step in laying the groundwork for a strong foundation starts now!

Take action before the end of the day, and then, with confidence, move on to the next chapter of your journey.

∞∞§∞∞

4

Nurturing the Parenting Mindset During Pregnancy

"**P**regnancy is a process that invites you to surrender to the unseen force behind all Life"_Jody Ford.

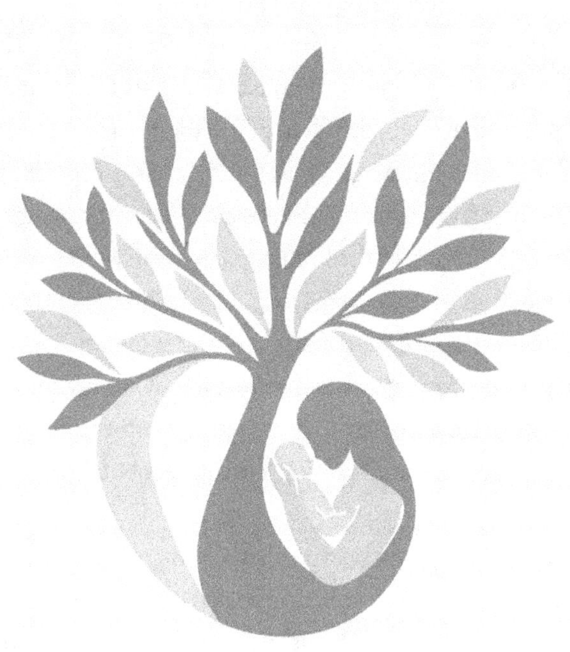

Let's start today with a Positive Mindset. I need your participation of 101% for your Little one who is waiting for a Healthy mindset fluid.

As we learned in our first chapter, research has proven that a child born with their parents' proper planning and mindset is more intelligent than a child born without adequate parental mindset or planning.

Perfect preparation and the right attitude can make your child a real-life superhero. Ready to unlock the potential of your future genius? It all starts with a bit of planning and a positive mindset!

As we understand in our last chapter, Nurturing the parenting mindset during pregnancy is a bit like planting seeds in a garden. You're preparing the soil, providing the proper nutrients, and patiently tending to the growth of positive thoughts and emotions.

Imagine your mind as a garden bed and each positive thought as a seed. Nurturing the parenting mindset involves consciously planting thoughts of joy, love, and confidence. It's about caring for your mental well-being, just like you would water and care for growing plants.

Consider this: Your mind is like a canvas, and during pregnancy, you're painting a picture of the kind of parent you want to be. Nurturing the parenting mindset is choosing bright and vibrant colors and creating a canvas filled with optimism, patience, and wonder.

It's similar to preparing a cozy nest for a new family member. Just as you might decorate a nursery with care and attention, nurturing the parenting mindset is about creating a positive mental space for yourself and your baby.

So, nurturing the parenting mindset during pregnancy is like being a gentle gardener, planting seeds of positivity and tending to the emotional landscape, ensuring a healthy and vibrant mental environment for both you and your growing family.

Let's Go through A Story that explains this topic better..

A couple named Lila and Oliver lived in a Beautiful village surrounded by meadows and gentle hills. They were on the brink of a new chapter in their lives as they eagerly anticipated the arrival of their first child. However, they understood that preparing for parenthood went beyond physical preparations; it required nurturing the right mindset.

As Lila's belly grew with the promise of a new life, she and Oliver embarked on a journey of cultivating a positive and nurturing parenting mindset. They believed the mindset they nurtured during pregnancy would lay the foundation for a loving and supportive family.

They began by creating a serene space in their home. Soft colors, cozy blankets, and calming music filled the air. In this sanctuary, Lila and Oliver would spend time together, talking to their unborn child, sharing dreams, and envisioning the joyful moments that awaited them.

Lila was an avid reader and immersed herself in books that focused on positive parenting techniques and mindful practices. She discovered the power of visualization and began to create a mental picture of the kind of parent she aspired to be. Oliver, a lover of nature, planted a small garden, symbolizing the growth and blossoming of their family.

They attended parenting classes where they learned about the importance of communication, setting intentions, and fostering a strong connection with their child. Lila and Oliver practiced mindfulness exercises, embracing the present moment and preparing their hearts for the beautiful chaos of parenthood.

As they ventured into the community, they sought guidance from experienced parents and elders who shared stories of resilience, laughter, and the profound joy of parenthood. These stories became beacons of inspiration, illuminating the path ahead.

Lila and Oliver also took the time to reflect on their childhoods, drawing from the positive experiences that shaped them. They acknowledged that parenting wasn't about perfection but creating a nurturing environment where their child could flourish.

They sat under a canopy of stars during quiet evenings, sharing their hopes and fears. They wrote letters to their unborn child, expressing their unconditional love and commitment. These letters, placed in a special box, would become a treasure chest of memories for their family.

As the day approached for their family to welcome a new member, Lila and Oliver felt a profound sense of readiness. Their home, filled with love and thoughtful preparation, was a testament to their nurtured mindset during pregnancy.

When their little one finally arrived, Lila and Oliver embraced parenthood with open hearts. The nurturing mindset they had cultivated became the guiding light, helping them navigate the sleepless nights, the first steps, and the countless moments of wonder.

Years passed, and their home echoed with the laughter of a growing family. Lila and Oliver, now seasoned parents, looked back on their journey with gratitude. The mindset they had nurtured during pregnancy had become the heartbeat of their family, a melody of love, patience, and the unwavering belief in the beauty of parenthood.

In the quiet moments, as they watched their child play in the garden, Lila and Oliver knew that the seeds they had planted during pregnancy had flourished into a garden of resilience, joy, and a deep connection that would blossom for generations.

And so, in their village nestled among meadows and hills, Lila, Oliver, and their little one lived a life infused with the magic of nurturing the parenting mindset. This story echoed the transformative power of intention, love, and the gentle whispers of preparation during the precious months of pregnancy.

It's Activity time,

Here is a simple activity that we are going to do right now.

Every morning, when you wake up with a big smile, and every night before you go to bed, write ten positive words for yourself to repeat.

That's it. Easy…?

There are two options for you.

1. You select any ten sentences from your end.
2. I will give you it, and you can choose from it.

"Step into the rhythm of your journey with joy and anticipation. This space is your canvas, and each sentence is a stroke of positivity, weaving a masterpiece of your path to motherhood. Let these words be your daily affirmation, resonating with the magic of new life. Embrace the beauty of this moment and let this table reflect the incredible journey you're on."

Fostering a positive mindset during pregnancy is crucial. Here are my ten positive sentences, especially for you.

1. "I am surrounded by love and support, creating a nurturing environment for my baby."
2. "Every day, my body becomes stronger and more capable of bringing new life into the world."
3. "I trust my body's wisdom to grow and nourish my baby in the healthiest way possible."
4. "Each kick and flutter reminds me of the miracle unfolding within me."
5. "I am calm, confident, and ready to embrace the journey of motherhood."
6. "My mind is filled with joy, gratitude, and anticipation for my baby's arrival."
7. "I radiate positivity and a peaceful and loving energy surrounds my baby."
8. "I am creating a deep and loving bond with my baby, even before their arrival."

9. "Every day brings me closer to holding my precious baby in my arms."

10. "I am a strong and resilient woman, capable of facing any challenges that come my way."

I'm here to deliver on my promise and give you even more - an extra 10, just for you...

11. "Embraced by the cocoon of love around me, each day brings my baby closer to my heart."

12. "My body, a symphony of strength, is orchestrating the beautiful crescendo of new life within."

13." In the dance of creation, my body is the canvas, painting a masterpiece of life and love."

14. "Tiny flutters echo the sweet melody of anticipation, a lullaby composed by my growing miracle."

15." In the quiet moments, I find serenity, knowing I am a vessel of calm for my baby's journey."

16. "My thoughts bloom like flowers in a garden, creating a fragrant tapestry of joy and positivity."

17. "With every beat of my heart, I send waves of love, wrapping my baby in a blanket of tranquility."

18. "Our connection, a celestial dance, weaves an unbreakable bond, setting the stage for a lifetime of love."

19. "In the hush of expectancy, I find peace, relishing the precious moments of becoming a mother."

20." As the days unfurl, I draw closer to the magical chapter when I cradle my little one in pure, unbridled joy."

∞∞∞§∞∞∞

5

Purification of Your Mind

"There is an old saying that if you want to fill your glass with holy water, first you have to empty the dirty water of the glass."

We all are a small part of the Ultimate Pure Energy we call God, so we all are pure souls, and there is no dought about it, but our habits and surrounding atmosphere make us impure. But don't worry, we are on the way to becoming pure, and even the impure word itself says, "I'm PURE."

Embark on the remarkable journey of "Mindful Pregnancy," where we explore the powerful transformation of cultivating a purified mind. In this chapter, we'll learn practices that not only benefit you but also create a calm and nurturing space for the growing life within.

Role of the Subconsiousmind during Pregnancy

Do you know that the working of one part of our body is still undiscovered entirely by our scientists? Mind how our mind works is still a topic of discovery for scientists.

Let's understand our mind, which our scientists have discovered to date.

Have you seen an Iceberg…? Most of us have probably seen one in the movie *'Titanic'*. Am I right? 10% Iceberg we can see, 90% we can't. Our mind's functionality looks the same.

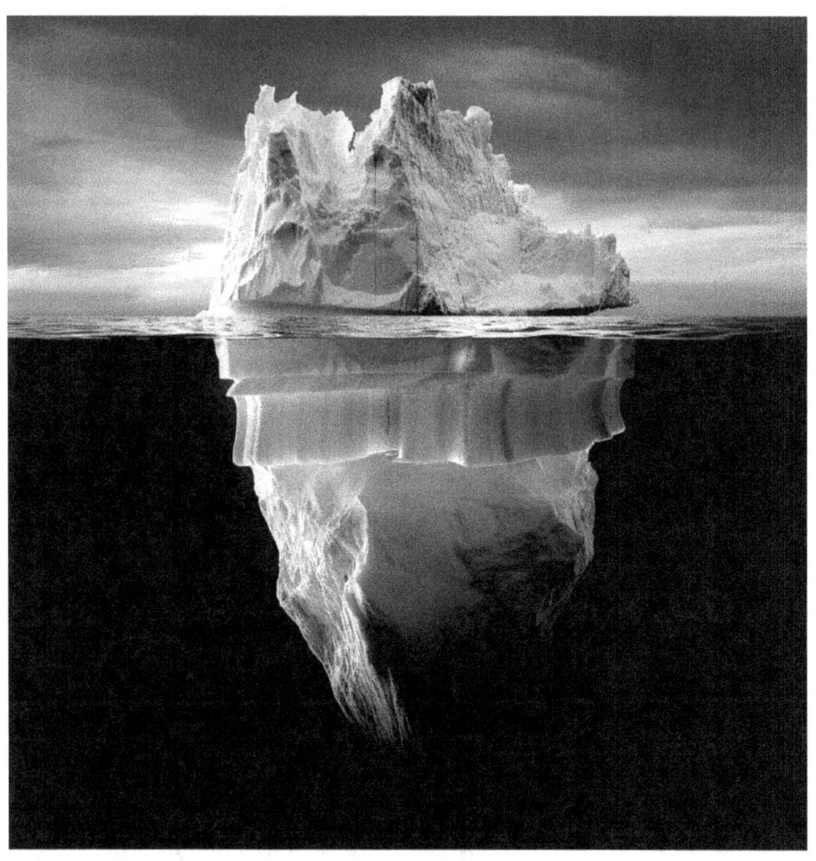

In standard language, our mind has two parts: conscious & subconscious.

A. Conscious mind

Certainly! The conscious mind is like the captain of a ship, steering and making decisions as we navigate through life. It's the part of our mind we're aware of, the thoughts and actions we actively choose and control. For example, when you decide to eat a healthy meal or go for a walk, that's your conscious mind at work.

Think of it as the tip of the Iceberg—the part that's visible above the water. It's responsible for logical thinking, problem-solving, and decision-making. When you're studying for an exam or planning your day, you're using your conscious mind to focus and make choices.

The bottom line is that our conscious mind charges our body when we are in a wake-up condition.

B. Sub Consiousmind

Let's dive into understanding the subconscious mind. Imagine it as the hidden depths below the ocean's surface. This expansive realm holds the memories, beliefs, and emotions that influence our behavior without realizing it.

Unlike the conscious mind, which is like the captain steering the ship, the subconscious mind is more like the crew working tirelessly behind the scenes. It's constantly processing information, storing memories, and influencing our thoughts and actions, often without conscious awareness.

For example, have you ever experienced a sudden feeling of fear or anxiety without knowing why? That could be your subconscious mind reacting to past experiences or deeply ingrained beliefs. It's also where habits, routines, and automatic responses are formed, like driving a car or tying your shoclaces without consciously thinking about it.

In essence, the subconscious mind is a powerhouse of information and influence, shaping our perceptions and behaviors in ways we may not fully understand. Understanding its role can empower us to tap into its potential and positively change our lives.

How does your subconscious mind help you during pregnancy?

Embarking on the journey of pregnancy is like setting sail on a thrilling adventure. Imagine your mind as a treasure map, with your subconscious serving as your trusty compass, guiding you through uncharted waters. Think of your subconscious as a hidden treasure trove, brimming with valuable insights and secrets waiting to be discovered. As an expectant mom, tapping into this inner wisdom can be your secret weapon for navigating pregnancy confidently and gracefully.

Understanding your subconscious is like unlocking a hidden vault of treasures. It allows you to unearth any fears or worries lurking beneath the surface, empowering you to face them head-on and transform them into sources of strength. But the magic doesn't stop there. Your subconscious also holds the key to staying positive throughout your pregnancy journey. By harnessing the power of positive thinking and visualization, you can turn challenges into opportunities for growth and resilience.

So, as you set sail on this extraordinary voyage, let your subconscious be your guiding star. Embrace the obscure with mental fortitude and interest, knowing that inside you lies the ability to explore any tempest and find the secret fortunes that anticipate.

During pregnancy, your subconscious mind significantly shapes your thoughts, emotions, and experiences. It operates like a hidden powerhouse within your brain, influencing your beliefs, attitudes, and behaviors without conscious awareness. Deep-seated fears or anxieties about childbirth, parenting, or your baby's health may reside in your subconscious, affecting your emotional well-being and overall state. These fears can manifest as stress, anxiety, or physical symptoms, potentially impacting your pregnancy and birth experience.

Contrastingly, cultivating a positive and empowered subconscious mindset can yield significant benefits during pregnancy. You tap into your inner strength, resilience, and intuition by nurturing positive thoughts, beliefs, and affirmations. This can result in reduced stress, improved emotional well-being, and positive pregnancy experiences.

Moreover, the subconscious mind is highly receptive to suggestion, making it a potent tool for visualization and manifestation. Techniques like guided imagery or positive affirmations can program your subconscious to focus on desired outcomes, fostering a smooth pregnancy, a healthy baby, or a positive birth experience. This approach can alleviate fears and promote calmness, confidence, and empowerment.

In summary, understanding and harnessing the power of your subconscious mind is crucial in shaping your pregnancy journey. By doing so, you cultivate a positive mindset, navigate challenges with resilience, and embrace the transformative experience of pregnancy with grace and confidence.

Let's understand your mind's power with a significant but small exercise.

Activity: Magnet Visualization

Before beginning the Activity, please take note of the following instructions:

1. **Visualization:** First, you have to understand the whole activity, and then, afterward, close your eyes. Once you understand the instructions clearly, you can see yourself performing the Activity in your mind.

2. **Trust the Process:** Your logical thinking may be challenged throughout the activity. Trust the process and focus solely on following the instructions provided.

3. **Duration:** This Activity will take only 2 minutes to complete, so

it's essential to dedicate this time to the exercise.

4. **Solitude:** Find a quiet and undisturbed space to carry out the Activity. Being alone will allow you to fully immerse yourself in the experience and gain maximum benefit from it.

Ready to experience the power of your mind?

1. Find a quiet, comfortable space where you won't be disturbed. Take a moment to relax and settle into a comfortable seated position. Close your eyes and take a few deep breaths to center yourself.

2. With your eyes closed, imagine that each of your hands is a powerful magnet, with one hand representing the North Pole and the other hand representing the South Pole. Feel the magnetic energy emanating from each hand as you visualize them in front of you.

3. Visualize the magnetic force between them, and continue and frequently repeat in your mind that both your hands have now become a powerful magnet. The magnetic force between them pulls them closer. Keep focusing on the image in your mind as you bring your hands closer and closer together.

4. As your hands come closer, please notice any sensations you feel between them. Notice if you sense a magnetic pull or any tingling sensations.

5. After a few moments, gently open your eyes and take a moment to reflect on your experience. Please take a look at any sensations or feelings that arose during the visualization.

6. **Trust the Process:** Remember that this Activity is about trusting the power of your mind and the process itself. Even if you didn't feel a physical sensation, trust that the visualization impacted your subconscious.

7. Be open to the experience and avoid the temptation to analyze or doubt the process. Instead, embrace the opportunity to connect with your subconscious mind and explore its potential.

8. **Repeat:** You can regularly repeat this visualization exercise to strengthen your connection with your subconscious mind and enhance your ability to manifest positive outcomes.

During this Activity, 95% of participants typically feel a magnetic sensation between their hands. For the remaining 5%, the inclination may be to analyze the Activity logically. Remember, your focus should be on trusting the process rather than scrutinizing its mechanics. Rest assured, the experience will unfold naturally.

Let's try another experience with the same hand, which will force you to rely on the visualization power of your brain.

Close your eyes and take a few deep breaths to center yourself. Position of both hands: straight from your elbow joint and in front of your eyes. Envision each of your hands as a strong magnet, both representing the north pole.Picture them in front of you, radiating magnetic energy.

Both hands became a north pole, visualizing the magnetic force pushing them apart. Visualize the magnetic force between them, and continue and frequently repeat in your mind that both your hands have become a powerful magnet of the north pole. The magnetic force between them pushes them. Keep focusing on the image in your mind.

Pay attention to any sensations or feelings between your hands. Notice if you feel a magnetic push or tingling between your hands.

When you're ready, gently open your eyes and take a moment to reflect on your experience.

Learnings from this Activity are that the true power lies within you, and tapping into your subconscious mind can unlock endless possibilities for growth and transformation.

Here, we discover the power of our thoughts. Positive thoughts yield positive actions, while negative thoughts lead to adverse outcomes. It's up to you to choose the thoughts you want to nurture for the well-being of your future child.

So now let's move ahead to our main Activity..

Subconscious Visualization

1. Find a quiet, comfortable space where you won't be disturbed.
2. Close your eyes and take several deep breaths to relax your body and calm your mind.
3. Visualize yourself in a serene setting, such as a peaceful garden or a secluded beach.
4. Imagine a glowing orb of light hovering above you, representing your subconscious mind. See it radiating with positive energy and vibrant colors.
5. As you focus on the glowing orb, allow any thoughts or emotions to arise naturally. Notice any fears, worries, or doubts lingering in your subconscious.
6. Now, visualize yourself releasing these negative thoughts and replacing them with empowering affirmations and beliefs. See them transforming into beams of light that radiate from the glowing orb and envelop you in a warm embrace.
7. Take a moment to bask in the glow of positivity and empowerment, feeling a sense of peace and reassurance wash over you.
8. When you're ready, gently bring your awareness back to the present moment. Open your eyes and take a few more deep breaths to ground yourself.
9. Reflect on your experience and any insights or revelations that

may have emerged during the visualization.

10. Consider incorporating this practice into your daily routine to connect with your subconscious mind and cultivate a positive mindset throughout your pregnancy.

Conclusion and Benefits of Subconscious Visualization

Subconscious visualization is a powerful practice that allows you to tap into the depths of your mind and harness its transformative potential. Engaging in this practice creates a sacred space for self-reflection, empowerment, and growth. Here are some key benefits of incorporating subconscious visualization into your pregnancy journey:

1. **Stress Reduction:** Subconscious visualization helps alleviate stress and anxiety by allowing you to release negative thoughts and emotions stored in your subconscious. By visualizing yourself letting go of fears and worries, you create space for relaxation and inner peace.

2. **Empowerment:** Through subconscious visualization, you can replace limiting beliefs with empowering affirmations and beliefs. You cultivate confidence, strength, and resilience by being surrounded by positive energy and vibrant colors.

3. **Connection with Baby:** Subconscious visualization allows you to connect with your baby more deeply. As you visualize yourself in a serene setting, you can also visualize your baby surrounded by love and protection, fostering a strong bond between you and your little one.

4. **Manifestation:** By visualizing positive outcomes and desired experiences, you can manifest them into reality. Subconscious visualization allows you to tap into the creative power of your mind and align your thoughts with your intentions, helping you manifest a smooth and joyful pregnancy journey.

5. **Self-Reflection:** Subconscious visualization encourages self-reflection and introspection, Enabling you to gain insights into your thoughts, emotions, and beliefs. By reflecting on your experiences during visualization, you can uncover hidden truths and discover new perspectives on your pregnancy journey.

Overall, subconscious visualization is a valuable tool for nurturing your mind, body, and spirit during pregnancy. By integrating this practice into your daily routine, you can cultivate a positive mindset, enhance your well-being, and embrace the transformative journey of motherhood with grace and confidence.

∞∞∞§∞∞∞

6

The Role of a Supportive Partner

"Having a baby is like falling in love again, both with your husband and your child"_Tina Brown.

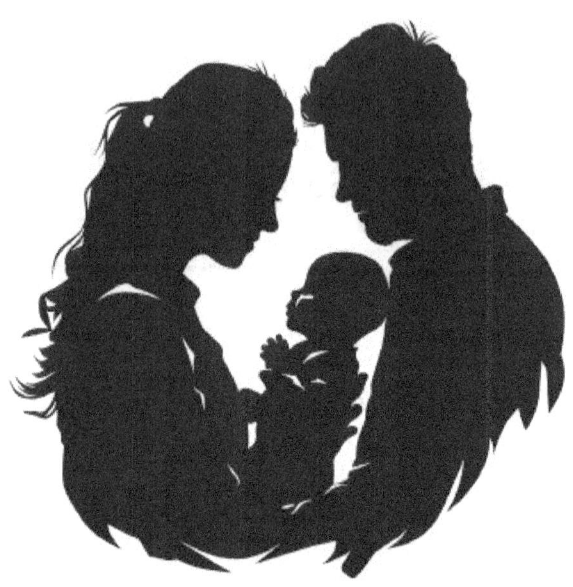

The role of a supportive partner is like having a reliable co-pilot on the journey of becoming a parent. Like in a good team, both partners play crucial roles, and having a supportive partner is like having someone who has your back and cheering you on.

Think of it as teamwork. A supportive partner listens when you want to share your thoughts and feelings about becoming a parent. They offer a helping hand when things get overwhelming and celebrate the exciting moments with you. It's about creating a solid partnership where you feel understood and supported.

Imagine you're on a tandem bike – both pedaling together towards the same destination. A supportive partner keeps the bike steady, helps with the uphill climbs, and shares the joy of cruising down the hills. In the journey to parenthood, a supportive partner is there to share the load, navigate challenges, and enjoy the beautiful moments together.

So, the role of a supportive partner is like having a teammate who is there for you, making the path to parenthood smoother and more enjoyable. It's a partnership filled with understanding, encouragement, and shared excitement.

This Activity is For your Loved One...
What's your First thought?
Aah.. this chapter is my Favourite... Isn't it?

Let's go to today's Activity...
The role of a supportive partner during pregnancy involves a range of responsibilities to provide emotional support, active involvement, and overall well-being for both the pregnant woman and the relationship.
Here are three important daily tasks a supportive partner can undertake :

1. **Emotional Connection:**

- **Task:** Check in on Emotions
- **Description:** Daily, actively inquire about the pregnant partner's emotions, concerns, and experiences. Listen attentively, express empathy, and offer reassurance. Creating a safe space for open communication fosters emotional connection and strengthens the bond between partners.

2. **Active Participation:**

- **Task:** Attend Prenatal Activities
- **Description:** Actively engage in prenatal activities, such as accompanying the pregnant partner to doctor's appointments, attending prenatal classes, or participating in birthing preparation exercises. It demonstrates active support, strengthens the partner's understanding of the pregnancy process, and fosters a sense of togetherness.

3. **Practical Support:**

- **Task:** Assist with Daily Tasks
- **Description:** Contribute to daily tasks and responsibilities, recognizing the physical changes and potential challenges the pregnant partner may face. I'd like to offer assistance with household chores, meal preparation, or other practical aspects to help ease stress and ensure a supportive environment. This daily support contributes to the overall well-being of both partners.

A supportive partner actively contributes to a positive and nurturing pregnancy experience by consistently incorporating these tasks into the daily routine. These actions not only strengthen the relationship but also create an environment where the pregnant woman feels valued, supported, and emotionally connected throughout the journey to parenthood.

Understanding Emotional Preparation

"A baby is something you carry inside you for nine months, in your arms for three years, and in your heart, until the day you die"_Mary Mason.

Understanding emotional preparation is like getting ready for a big journey. Still, instead of packing bags, you're getting your feelings and thoughts in order. It's about taking some time to think about how you feel about becoming a parent. Are you excited, nervous, or both? It's also about talking to your partner, sharing your thoughts, and listening to theirs.

Imagine this: Before going on a road trip, you'd check the weather, plan your route, and make sure your car is ready. Emotional preparation is like checking in with yourself and your partner before the adventure of parenthood. It's acknowledging your feelings, having open conversations, and ensuring you're both on the same page.

So, understanding emotional preparation is about pausing, looking inward, and having heart-to-heart talks as you prepare for the incredible journey of becoming parents.

Here's a beautiful story about Understanding Emotional Preparation.

Once upon a time, a couple named James and Rose lived in a small town. They were overjoyed to discover that they were going to become parents. Excitement filled their hearts, but soon, they realized that along with joy, there were moments of uncertainty and nervousness.

As they prepared for this new chapter in their lives, Rose and James decided to embark on a journey of emotional preparation. They attended prenatal classes, read books on parenting, and sought advice from experienced parents in their community. However, they soon realized that emotional preparation wasn't just about gaining knowledge; it was about understanding and embracing the emotions that parenthood brings.

One day, as they strolled through a serene park, Rose shared her worries about being a good mother. She expressed her fears of not living up to societal expectations and making mistakes. James, being the supportive partner he was, held her hand and said, "Rose, emotional preparation is not about being perfect; it's about being present and learning from the journey. We're in this together, and that's what matters."

They decided to create a "Parenting Journal," a shared space where they could jot down their feelings, hopes, and fears. Every week, they set aside time to sit together and discuss their entries. Through this practice, they found solace in each other's company. They discovered that vulnerability and open communication were the pillars of emotional preparation.

As Rose's pregnancy progressed, so did their emotional bond. They attended prenatal yoga classes, practiced mindfulness together, and shared a quiet moment each day to connect with their unborn child. The emotional rollercoaster became a shared adventure, with both Rose and James finding strength in their unity.

When the day finally arrived to welcome their baby into the world, Rose and James felt many emotions—excitement, nervousness, and overwhelming love. In the delivery room, as they held their newborn in their arms, they knew that their journey of emotional preparation had laid a strong foundation for the beautiful moments of parenthood.

Activity Time: Cherishing Moments Together

Life's fast pace often leaves little room for connection. Today, carve out a precious 30 minutes with your partner. Amid the daily hustle, set aside distractions – no phones, no screens, just the two of you.

Here's Your Simple Activity:

A. Plan Your Journey:

- Sit down together and reflect on your journey, embracing the beautiful opportunity of parenthood.
- Choose a dedicated time, free from the buzz of technology, and reserve it exclusively for each other.

B. Daily Highlights:

- Share the good things that happened in your day. Celebrate the joys and victories, no matter how small.
- If you have any more challenges, please discuss how to navigate them, ensuring a brighter tomorrow.

C. Checklist for Harmony:

- You can use a checklist to organize your thoughts and goals for the day.
- Please make sure you follow your unique route for a smoother and happier journey.

D. Work Matters:

- If you're working, discuss any challenges or highlights in your professional life.
- Support each other by identifying areas of growth and success.

This activity is more than a routine; it's a shared moment of reflection and planning. Let the warmth of your connection guide you, and relish in the joy of building a foundation for your growing family.

∞∞∞§∞∞∞

7

Food: Nourishing the Miracle Within

"**G**rowing a baby is like crafting a masterpiece; every nutrient, every meal, every bite is a stroke of brilliance."

Food is a big topic, but here we understand which food is most important during pregnancy for both the mother and child.

Pregnancy brings not only the joy of anticipation but also the responsibility of nurturing a new life. It's important to think carefully about what you eat on this journey. Your body is now a home for two, and the food and beverages you consume have a significant impact on the general health and development of your unborn child.

Let us understand more deeply. Here, we know four main parts as a section.

A. Nourishing Your Baby's Growth

B. Importance of Protein-Rich Diet

C. Importance of Hydration

D. The Role of Supplements

A. Nourishing Your Baby's Growth

In this Section, we embark on a journey through the world of nutrition, exploring the key elements essential for your baby's healthy development during pregnancy. Let's delve into the three crucial nutrients – folic acid, iron, and calcium – and understand why they are the building blocks for your baby's growth.

A.1 Folic Acid:

First on our list of topics to research is folic acid, a necessary nutrient that helps shield developing children's spine and brain against birth abnormalities. Broccoli, kale, and other leafy greens are good providers of folic acid. Explore the world of colorful salads and nutrient-dense smoothies to include these greens to your diet with ease.

A.2 Iron:

Iron is the next food on our nutritional trip. Iron is necessary for the production of red blood cells, which helps to avoid anemia in pregnant women. Rich sources of iron include fowl, beans, lentils, and lean meats. Learn how to prepare delectable dishes with these iron-rich foods to guarantee a balanced and healthy diet.

A.3 Calcium:

As we proceed, calcium takes the spotlight for its crucial role in developing your baby's bones and teeth. Dairy products like milk, yogurt, and cheese are classic calcium sources. However, if you prefer plant-based options, fortified plant milk, leafy greens, and nuts can provide the calcium your baby needs.

Managing your diet while expecting may be a happy and rewarding experience. The goal of this chapter is to arm you with the knowledge you need to make wise decisions and guarantee that both you and your unborn child get the nutrition you need for a healthy and happy pregnancy. Together, let's go off on this fulfilling journey.

B. Importance of Protein-Rich Diet During Pregnancy:

A protein-rich diet is crucial during pregnancy as it plays a pivotal role in the mother's and baby's growth and development. Proteins are:

- The building blocks of life.
- Contributing to the formation of tissues.
- Organs.
- Essential enzymes.

Here's why a protein-rich diet is of utmost importance:

B.1 Cellular Growth and Repair:

- Proteins are essential for the growth and repair of cells, ensuring that both the mother's body and the developing baby receive the necessary nutrients for optimal development.

B.2 Organ and Tissue Development:

- During pregnancy, the baby's organs and tissues are rapidly developing. Proteins provide the necessary amino acids that contribute to forming these vital structures, promoting overall health and functionality.

B.3 Supporting the Immune System:

- Protein is essential to the immune system's capacity to defend the body against illnesses and infections. An immune system that is robust is necessary to safeguard both the developing fetus and the expectant mother.

B.4 Blood Volume Expansion:

- As pregnancy progresses, blood volume increases to meet the growing demands of the developing baby. Proteins play a role in maintaining adequate blood volume, supporting proper circulation and oxygen delivery to both the mother and the baby.

B.5 Preventing Protein Deficiency Issues:

- Preterm delivery, low birth weight, and poor brain development are just a few of the issues that can result from consuming insufficient protein during pregnancy. A diet high in protein reduces these risks and encourages a safe pregnancy.

Let's now look at some fantastic protein sources that you may include in your regular meals:

B.5.1 Lean Meats:
Add fish, chicken, and lean beef or pig chops to your diet. These are great places to get high-grade protein.

B.5.2 Dairy Products:
Milk, yogurt, and cheese are protein-rich and provide essential calcium for bone health.

B.5.3 Eggs:
All the necessary amino acids needed for good health are present in eggs, making them a flexible source of protein.

B.5.4 Legumes:
Beans, lentils, and chickpeas are plant-based protein sources, offering

fiber and various nutrients.

B.5.5 Nuts and Seeds:

Almonds, peanuts, chia seeds, and sunflower seeds are nutrient-dense options for boosting protein intake.

B.5.6 Tofu and Soy Products:

Tofu, tempeh, and soy-based products are suitable alternatives for vegetarians, providing ample protein.

B.5.7 Quinoa:

As a complete protein, quinoa is a whole grain that contains all of the necessary amino acids.

Encouraging you to incorporate different foods high in protein into your regular meals guarantees that they fulfill your nutritional needs and supports a healthy pregnant journey.

C. Importance of Hydration During Pregnancy:

Since it directly affects the health and well-being of the expecting woman and the growing baby, maintaining proper hydration is crucial throughout pregnancy. Many physiological processes depend on maintaining adequate hydration. The following are the reasons why hydration is of utmost importance:

C.1 Optimal Blood Volume and Circulation:

- Adequate hydration supports blood volume expansion, ensuring a healthy circulation system. It is vital for transporting nutrients, oxygen, and hormones to the developing baby.

C.2 Amniotic Fluid Production:

- Amniotic fluid surrounds and protects the baby in the womb. Sufficient hydration contributes to the production and maintenance of amniotic fluid, providing a cushion for the baby and facilitating their movement.

C.3 Temperature Regulation:

- Hydration helps regulate body temperature, preventing overheating, especially during pregnancy when the body's natural cooling mechanisms may be more challenging to maintain.

C.4 Prevention of Dehydration-Related Complications:

- Constipation, premature contractions, urinary tract infections, and other problems can result from dehydration during pregnancy. Keeping enough water in your body lowers your chance of developing these problems.

C.5 Digestive Health:

- Drinking enough water supports proper digestion and helps prevent constipation, a common concern during pregnancy. It ensures the smooth absorption of nutrients essential for both the mother and the baby.

C.6 Reducing Swelling and Discomfort:

- Pregnancy-related symptoms like swelling and pain can be lessened by staying hydrated. Overall comfort is supported, and physiological fluid equilibrium is preserved.

C.7 Energy Levels and Fatigue Reduction:

- Dehydration can contribute to feelings of fatigue. Staying well-hydrated supports energy levels, allowing the expectant mother to cope with the physical demands of pregnancy more effectively.

C.8 Kidney Function and Toxin Elimination:

- Proper hydration supports kidney function, aiding in the elimination of waste products and toxins. It is crucial for both maternal and fetal health.

C.9 To ensure optimal hydration during pregnancy:

- Drink an adequate amount of water throughout the day.
- Consume hydrating foods like fruits and vegetables.
- Limit caffeinated and sugary beverages, as they may contribute to dehydration.

Encouraging expectant mothers to prioritize hydration is a simple yet powerful way to support a healthy pregnancy journey.

D. The Role of Supplements During Pregnancy:

A woman's pregnancy is a crucial time in her life as it requires extra nutrition to support the growth and development of the unborn child. Good nutrition starts with a well-balanced diet, but some supplements are essential to make sure the mother and the infant are getting enough food. This is a thorough analysis of the essential vitamins that are advised during pregnancy. In our first section, we touched on a few of them; now, let's delve further.

D.1 Folic Acid (Folate):

- **Role:** Essential for neural tube development, reducing the risk of congenital disabilities.
- **Food Sources:** Leafy greens, legumes, fortified cereals.
- **Supplement Recommendation:** Typically started before conception and continued during the first trimester.

D.2 Iron:

- **Role:** Supports the increased production of red blood cells to prevent anemia in both the mother and baby.
- **Food Sources:** Lean meats, beans, spinach.
- **Supplement Recommendation:** Often prescribed if dietary intake is insufficient.

D.3 Calcium:

- **Role:** Critical for the development of the baby's bones and teeth.
- **Food Sources:** Dairy products, fortified plant-based milk, leafy greens.
- **Supplement Recommendation:** This is important for women with lactose intolerance or inadequate dietary calcium.

D.4 Vitamin D:

- **Role:** Supports calcium absorption, which is crucial for bone health.

- **Food Sources:** Fatty fish, fortified dairy, exposure to sunlight.
- **Supplement Recommendation:** Often recommended, especially in regions with limited sunlight.

D.5 Omega-3 Fatty Acids:

- **Role:** Supports the development of the baby's brain and eyes.
- **Food Sources:** Fatty fish (e.g., salmon), flaxseeds, walnuts.
- **Supplement Recommendation:** Considered for those with limited fish intake.

D.6 Iodine:

- **Role:** Vital for the baby's brain development.
- **Food Sources:** Iodized salt, seafood.
- **Supplement Recommendation:** This is important, especially for those with low dietary iodine.

D.7 Vitamin B12:

- **Role:** Supports nerve function and the formation of red blood cells.
- **Food Sources:** Animal products, fortified foods.
- **Supplement Recommendation:** Essential for vegetarian or vegan mothers.

D.8 Vitamin C:

- **Role:** Aids in the absorption of non-heme iron from plant-based sources.
- **Food Sources:** Citrus fruits, strawberries, bell peppers.

You must consult your doctors before starting supplements, as individual needs may vary. The right combination of a balanced diet and supplements ensures comprehensive nutritional support for a healthy pregnancy.

∞∞§∞∞

8

Yogic Serenity - Navigating Pregnancy through Yoga

"**In the gentle flow of yoga, find the serenity to navigate the beautiful journey of pregnancy. Let each pose be a prayer, nurturing your body and soul as you prepare to welcome new life.**"

Yoga is a comprehensive discipline that has thousands of years of history and its roots in ancient India. Achieving balance and harmony in the body, mind, and spirit includes physical postures (asanas), breathing exercises (pranayama), meditation, and ethical precepts.

The Sanskrit word "yuj," which means to connect or combine, is where the term "yoga" originates. Enhancing general wellbeing and self-awarenessentails integrating the physical, mental, and spiritual facets of the person.

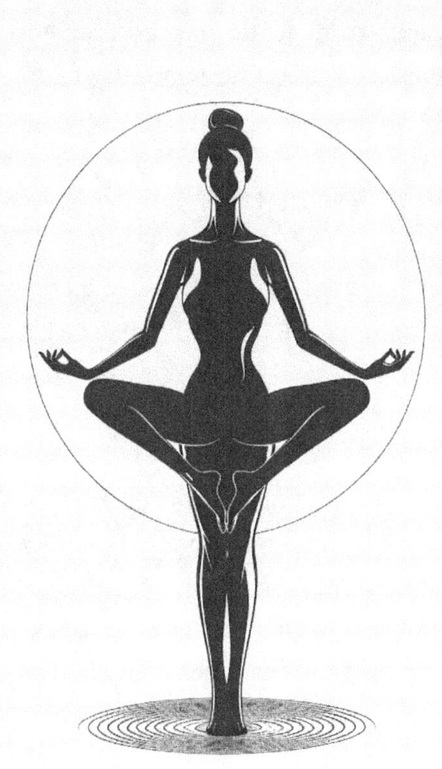

Nowadays, yoga has become famous worldwide as a form of exercise and relaxation. Numerous physical and psychological advantages are provided by it, such as enhanced flexibility, strength, balance, posture, and reduced stress. Frequent yoga practice can also help cultivate inner quiet and tranquility, increase awareness, and improve focus.

Yoga may be practiced in many different forms, including Hatha, Vinyasa, Ashtanga, Kundalini, and more, and is usually done on a mat. Though every style has a different focus and order of poses, they all aim to integrate the mind, body, and breath.

It's important to note that yoga is your personal journey, and you can adapt the practice to suit your needs and abilities. Many yoga classes are available, ranging from gentle and restorative to more vigorous and challenging, making it accessible to people of different ages, fitness levels, and backgrounds.

Pregnancy can bring about a number of benefits from yoga. In order to guarantee a safe and successful practice, it is advised that everyone interested in practicing yoga begin under the supervision of a certified instructor. This person can offer appropriate teaching and alignment cues.

Prenatal Yoga,

Prenatal yoga is specially made for expectant mothers and helps with strength, flexibility, and relaxation. Breathing techniques that are helpful during childbirth are frequently included.

Prenatal yoga promotes flexibility, relaxation, and general well-being, among other advantages for expectant mothers. The following yoga positions are often regarded as safe to perform while pregnant:

- **Mountain Pose (Tadasana):** Helps improve posture and balance.
- **Cat-Cow Stretch (Marjaryasana-Bitilasana):** Enhances flexibility in the spine and helps alleviate back pain.
- **Warrior II (Virabhadrasana II):** Strengthens the legs and opens the hips, promoting stamina.
- **Tree Pose (Vrikshasana):** Enhances balance and concentration while strengthening the legs.
- **Bound Angle Pose (Baddha Konasana):** Opens the hips and groin, relieving tight muscles.
- **Child's Pose (Balasana):** A resting pose that helps release tension in the back and shoulders.
- **Legs Up the Wall Pose (Viparita Karani):** Promotes serenity and lessens leg edema.

- **Puppy Pose (Uttana Shishosana):** Stretches the spine and shoulders gently.
- **Modified Triangle Pose (Trikonasana):** A safe way to stretch the sides of the body and open the hips.
- **Corpse Pose (Savasana):** A relaxation pose to end the practice, focusing on deep breathing and calming the mind.

Always consult a certified prenatal yoga instructor before starting any yoga practice during pregnancy. They can guide modifications and ensure the safety of both the mother and the baby.

Let's explore more parts of yoga.

During pregnancy, it's essential to prioritize safe exercises and promote overall well-being. Here are some recommended types of exercises for pregnant women:

- **Walking:** A simple and low-impact exercise that can be adapted to various fitness levels. It helps maintain cardiovascular health.
- **Swimming:** This low-impact exercise supports the weight of the growing belly. It's gentle on the joints and provides a full-body workout.
- **Pilates:** Emphasizes the need for core strength, especially during pregnancy. It is possible to customize Pilates workouts specifically for expecting moms.
- **Stationary Cycling:** Riding a stationary bike is a low-impact way to increase your heart rate without putting stress on the joints.
- **Prenatal Aerobics:** Tailored aerobics classes for pregnant women are designed to keep you fit while considering the changes in your body.
- **Strength Training:** Muscle tone can be preserved with the use of resistance bands or light weights. Keep your form correct and steer

clear of hard lifting.

Prior to beginning any workout regimen while pregnant, always get medical advice. Based on each person's unique health and pregnancy circumstances, they may offer tailored advice.

∞∞§∞∞

9

GarbhSanskar - Cultivating a Positive Womb Environment

What is Garbh Sanskar?

Garbh Sanskar, rooted in Indian culture, is a traditional practice that emphasizes the fetus's well-being during pregnancy. "Garbh" means womb, and "Sanskar" refers to the process of imparting values or refining.

Understanding Garbh Sanskar

Garbh Sanskar is a set of practices and rituals designed to create a positive environment for the unborn child, both physically and spiritually. The belief is that the mental and emotional state of the mother directly influences the development of the baby in the womb.

Garbhsanskar, also known as prenatal education or fetal education, is an ancient Indian practice that focuses on the overall development of the fetus during pregnancy.

It is based on the belief that a positive and nurturing environment and experiences during pregnancy can benefit the unborn child's physical, mental, and spiritual well-being.

Let's understand with an example...

As we talked early in our book, we thought about how enormous icebergs are, with most of their mass hidden underwater. Well, a baby's brain is a bit like that – about 80% of its growth happens when the baby is inside the mom's tummy, like the hidden part of the Iceberg. The rest, around 20%, occurs after the baby is born.

Here's the exciting part: the mom has a significant role in shaping that hidden 80%. This book explores ways to help your baby's brain grow during this best time. Here are Important elements of Garbha Sanskar,

Conscious Pregnancy:

- **Positive Environment:** Garbha Sanskar emphasizes creating a positive and harmonious environment for the expecting mother. This includes fostering positive thoughts, emotions, and surroundings.

Diet and Nutrition:

- **Sattvic Diet:** Researchers recommend a clean, nutrient-dense, and easily digested diet. Fresh produce, whole grains, and dairy products are included in this group. It is often believed that a mother's diet has a direct effect on the physical and mental health of her fetus.

Moral and Ethical Values:

- **Inculcating Values:** Garbha Sanskar encourages pregnant women to engage in activities that promote moral and ethical values. This includes exposure to uplifting literature, music, and positive influences.

Meditation and Spiritual Practices:

- **Meditation and Prayer:** Believers hold that practices like meditation, chanting, and prayer positively impact the mental and spiritual development of the fetus. These practices are believed to foster a sense of tranquility and spiritual connection.

Reading and Listening:

- **Positive Content:** Reading and listening to positive and spiritually uplifting content during pregnancy is beneficial. This includes sacred texts, stories, and music that convey positive messages.

Ayurvedic Therapies:

- **Herbal Support:** Ayurvedic principles are often incorporated, including using specific herbs and oils to support the physical well-being of the mother and the developing child.

Yoga and Physical Exercises:

- **Gentle Yoga:** Doing gentle yoga and prenatal exercises is encouraged to maintain physical health and flexibility and promote relaxation.

Bonding with the Unborn Child:

- **Communication:** Communication and bonding activities are vital to establish a connection with the unborn child. This involves talking, singing, and expressing love to the baby.

Avoiding Negative Influences:

- **Limiting Stress:** Garbha Sanskar advises pregnant women to avoid stressful situations, negative influences, and negative emotions, which are believed to impact the child's temperament.

Panchakarma:

- **Detoxification:** In some cases, Ayurvedic detoxification processes known as Panchakarma may be recommended for the mother to ensure a healthy and toxin-free environment for the baby.

∞∞∞§∞∞∞

10

Exploring Music Therapy-Harmonies of Motherhood

"**M**usic can change the world because it can change people." - Bono

Symphony of Serenity - Elevating Pregnancy with Harmonious Melodies

In the enchanting realm of pregnancy, where emotions weave a delicate tapestry, we delve into the magical world of music therapy. Just as a symphony orchestrates myriad notes into a harmonious masterpiece, music has the transformative power to shape our emotional landscape. This chapter invites you to embrace the therapeutic embrace of music during this precious journey.

The Power of Sound

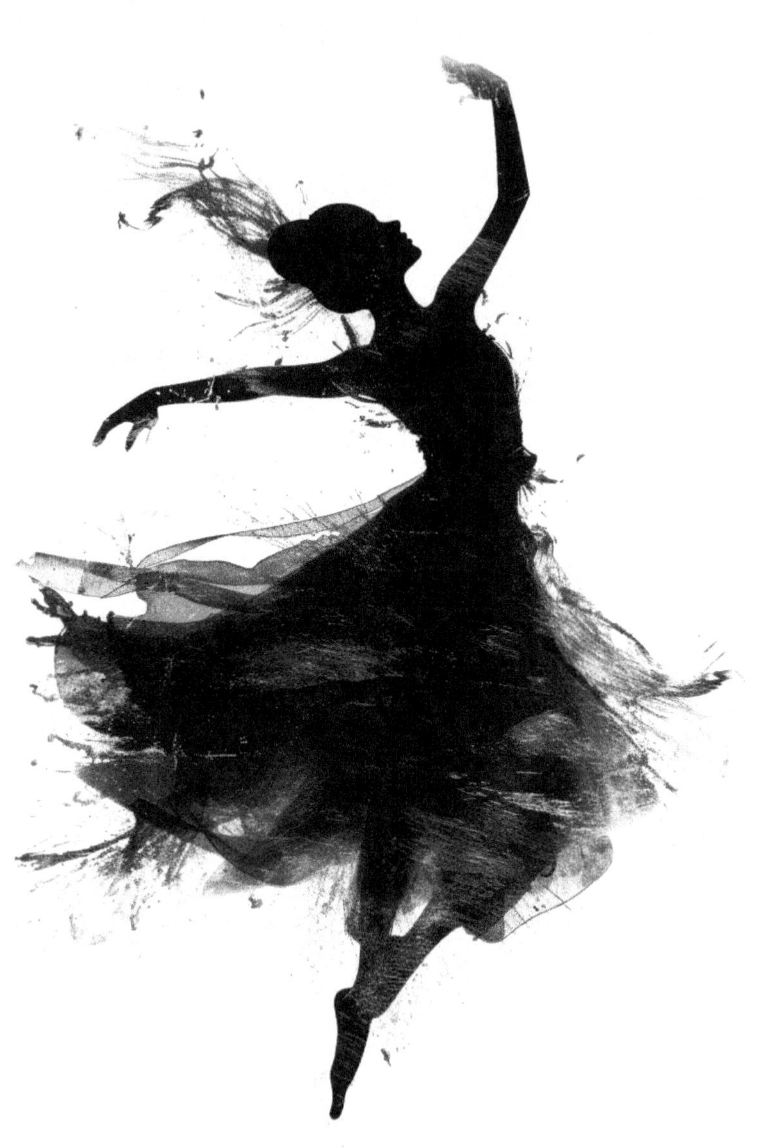

Unravel the profound impact of sound vibrations on our emotional canvas. Explore the interconnections between music and the tapestry of human emotions, setting the stage for a deeper exploration into the world of music therapy.

A. Benefits of Music Therapy During Pregnancy:

A.1 Stress Reduction:

- Discover how the gentle strains of soothing melodies can act as a balm for the soul, alleviating the strains of stress and anxiety.
- Embark on a journey through real-life testimonials, unveiling music's transformative power in easing pregnancy burdens.

A.2 Emotional Connection:

- Delve into the emotional symphony between a mother and her unborn child, understanding how carefully chosen tunes can enhance this profound connection.
- Uncover the ways in which music becomes a conduit for shared emotions, fostering a unique bond that transcends words.

A.3 Promoting Relaxation:

- Navigate through genres and rhythms tailor-made for relaxation, creating a personalized playlist that resonates with your tranquility.
- Learn techniques for seamlessly integrating music into daily routines, infusing moments of calm and serenity.

A.4 Physical Well-being:

- Unearth the potential impact of music on physical health during pregnancy, exploring its role in promoting overall well-being.

- Engage in gentle movement and dance activities accompanied by melodies that celebrate the beauty of your changing body.

A.5 Creating Your Musical Sanctuary:

Crafting a serene haven at home is an art. Discover tips for curating an ambiance where music becomes an elixir for your soul. From ambient lighting to selecting the perfect acoustics, this Section guides you in creating a haven where every note resonates with peace.

B. Tips for Incorporating Music Therapy,

Elevate your experience with practical tips on seamlessly integrating music therapy into your daily routine. From curated playlists for different moods to exploring diverse musical genres, discover the art of weaving music into the fabric of your pregnancy.

As we reach the crescendo of this musical sojourn, reflect on the symphony of emotions and well-being that music has unfurled. This chapter is an ode to the transformative power of harmonious melodies, inviting you to dance to the rhythm of your heart and relish the sonorous beauty of pregnancy.

In this symphony of serenity, let the melodic strains of music become the soundtrack to your pregnancy, creating a cherished harmony that resonates through every beat of your journey.

Activity

So, are you ready for today's Activity? Believe me, this Activity is your favorite Activity. Let's Dive In!

Close your eyes and take a deep breath. Today's Activity is a symphony for both of you and your little one—a celebration of the miraculous bond you share.

Activity: A Musical Odyssey

Choose Your Anthem:

Select a piece of music that resonates with positivity and uplifts your spirit. Whether it's a favorite song or a motivational speech, let it be a melody that fills the room with joy.

Positive Vibes Only:

Your baby is soaking in every note, so let the music be a cascade of positivity. Avoid any tunes that carry a hint of sadness; this is a time for joyous melodies that will set the stage for a positive mindset.

Connect Through Sound:

As you listen, feel the vibrations of the music and envision them wrapping around you and your baby. Imagine the notes forming a cocoon of warmth and inspiration, creating an environment of pure serenity.

Dance to the Rhythm of Love:

If you feel the rhythm moving you, sway gently to the music. Let the melodies spark a dance between you and your baby, a beautiful expression of the love you share.

Reflect and Rejoice:

After the music fades away, please take a moment to reflect on the emotions it stirred within you. Journal your thoughts or share the experience with your partner; cherish this special connection you're fostering with your little one.

Remember, this isn't just music; it's a powerful tool to shape a positive and uplifting environment for your growing miracle. Enjoy this musical journey of love and connection!

∞∞∞§∞∞∞

11

Meditation Moments - Connecting with Your Inner Self

"In the silence of meditation, the mother finds her strength, her patience, and her inner peace to navigate the journey of motherhood."

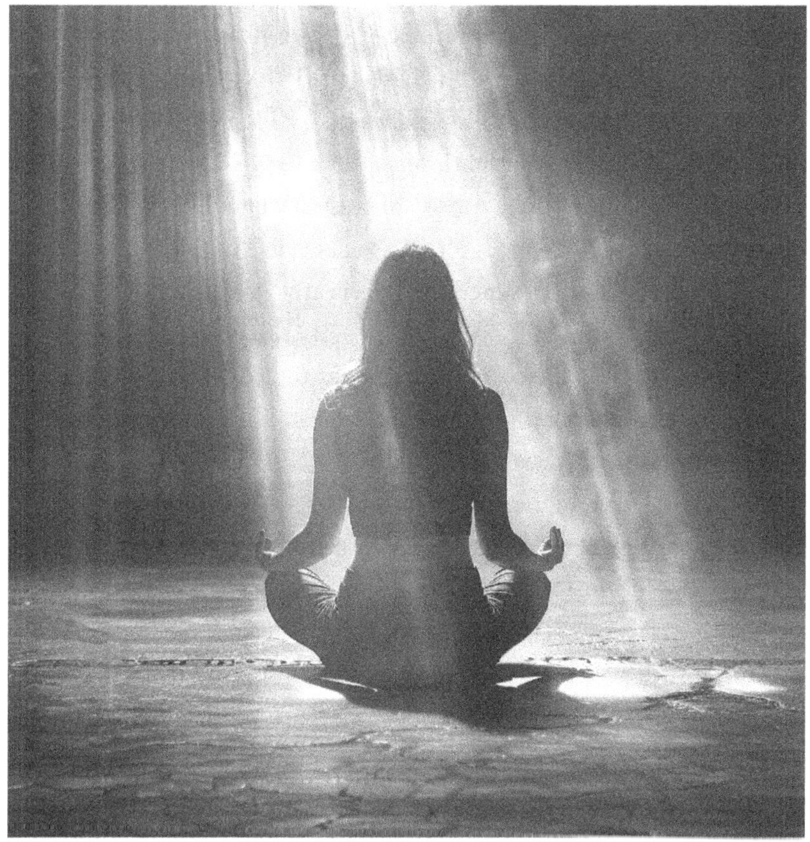

The Essence of Meditation - A Guide for Expectant Mothers

As you have understood our mind in past chapters, now you are aware of your mind's capacity, and it's time to use your brain correctly.

Let's go deeper in your brain.

Frequencies of Our Mind

The human mind operates at various frequencies, each associated with different states of consciousness and cognitive functions. Here are the main brainwave frequencies and their corresponding mind states. This information is only for knowledge purposes.

- **Beta (12-30 Hz):** This frequency range is associated with wakefulness and active mental engagement. Beta waves dominate ordinary waking consciousness, including problem-solving, decision-making, and focused attention.
- **Alpha (8-12 Hz):** Alpha waves are present when the mind is relaxed but still alert. This state is often associated with a calm and peaceful mind, such as during meditation, creative visualization, or light relaxation.
- **Theta (4-8 Hz):** Theta waves are linked to deep relaxation, creativity, and the subconscious mind. They occur during deep meditation, visualization, daydreaming, and REM sleep. Theta states are often associated with increased intuition, insight, and creativity.
- **Delta (0.5-4 Hz):** The slowest brainwave frequency, or delta waves, are most frequently connected to profound sleep and unconsciousness. They are essential for rejuvenation, bodily repair, and restful sleep.
- **Gamma (30-100 Hz):** Gamma waves are the fastest brainwave frequency associated with higher cognitive functions, such as memory recall, perception, and consciousness. They are also linked to moments of insight, heightened focus, and peak mental performance.

Each of these brainwave frequencies plays a vital role in regulating various aspects of cognitive function, emotional states, and overall mental well-being. Balancing and harmonizing these frequencies through practices like meditation, mindfulness, and relaxation techniques can help promote optimal mental health and cognitive function.

In this, Alpha waves (8-12 Hz) are a state when we reach during meditation. As our earlier chapter explains, positive affirmation is God's Word for your Baby. You must do a meditation once in a day.

Now, let's go Deep into our main Topic.

What is Meditation?

At its essence, meditation is a practice that invites you to explore the tranquility within. It's an inward journey, away from the external chatter, to discover the calm sanctuary within each of us. For the expectant mother, it becomes a gentle yet powerful tool to navigate the waves of pregnancy.

Understanding Meditation :

Picture meditation as a serene lake – still, reflective, and undisturbed. In the same way, meditation encourages a state of inner stillness. It's not about emptying the mind but observing thoughts without judgment, creating a space for peace to blossom.

Starting the Journey :

Embarking on the Meditation Journey:

Start with the fundamentals if you're new to meditation. Locate a peaceful, comfortable area where you won't be bothered. Shut your eyes, take a few deep breaths, and sit or lie down in a comfortable posture. Turn your focus within and let the outside world slip away.

Simple Breath Awareness:

One basic method of meditation is to pay attention to your breath. Take note of how each breath in and breath out feels. As ideas start to cross your mind, and they always will, gently bring it back to the breath. This exercise helps you become more conscious in addition to grounding yourself in the here and now.

Benefits for You and Your Baby

Reducing Stress and Anxiety:

Even while it's a wonderful experience, being pregnant may also cause worry and anxiety. Meditation turns into a haven that provides relief from anxieties. Regular meditation may lower stress hormones and improve emotional health, according to research.

Connection with Your Baby:

As you delve into meditation, you create a sacred space for connection. Your baby, cocooned within, is sensitive to the vibrations of your emotions. A calm maternal mind becomes a haven, fostering a deep and harmonious bond between you and your little one.

Strengthening Emotional Well-Being:

Meditation is like a gentle balm for the emotional fluctuations that pregnancy may bring. It equips you with tools to navigate the emotional terrain, fostering a positive mindset and resilience in facing challenges.

Making it a Daily Practice

Integration into Daily Life:

Meditation's charm lies in its simplicity. It doesn't need hours of free time or a complicated setup. Begin with a short amount of time and then expand it until it becomes an important part of your daily routine. Find a calm moment before bed or in the morning that helps you feel at ease.

Creating Sacred Moments:

Think of meditation as creating sacred moments in your day. These moments, however brief, become anchors of tranquility. They are not just breaks but opportunities to nourish your mind, body, and the life growing within.

Importance of the Chapter:

Meditation, in its purest form, is a gift you offer to yourself and your baby. It's a journey of self-discovery, a path to tranquility amidst the beautiful chaos of pregnancy. As you embark on this exploration, may each breath become a melody of serenity, weaving a tapestry of peace for you and your little one.

Activity Time..

So, are sweet mothers ready to add a new and significant activity in your lives?

The good thing is you don't need any particular time for it. You can do it when you wake up or go to Bed.

Introduction:

Welcome to your daily meditation practice designed to nurture your mind, body, and spirit during this transformative journey of pregnancy. Find a quiet and comfortable space where you can fully relax and connect with your growing baby.

Let's begin… Meditation Process,

1. Settle into a Comfortable Position:
2. Sit or lie down in a comfortable position, ensuring your spine is straight and your body is fully supported. Close your eyes gently.
3. Deep Breathing:
4. Breathe deeply and slowly at first. Breathe deeply through your nose and feel your abdomen fill up completely. Breathe slowly through your lips, letting go of any tension or worry as you do so. Repeat these deep breathing exercises often, paying attention to your breathing rhythm.
5. Connect with Your Baby:

6. Place your hands gently on your abdomen, feeling the warmth and connection with your growing baby. Visualize a loving, golden light surrounding both you and your baby, creating a protective and nurturing cocoon.

7. Gratitude Meditation:

8. Take a moment to express gratitude for the miracle of pregnancy and the journey you are embarking on. Reflect on the incredible bond between you and your baby, feeling a deep appreciation for this precious gift of life.

9. Body Scan:

10. Slowly scan through your body from head to toe, bringing awareness to each area. With every breath, please pay attention to any tightness or pain in those locations and allow it to release. With each breath, nourish your body and your unborn child by sending them love and healing energy.

11. Affirmations:

12. Repeat positive affirmations tailored to pregnancy and motherhood. Affirm your strength, resilience, and capacity to nurture and care for your baby. Visualize a smooth and healthy pregnancy, trusting in your body's innate wisdom to support you every step of the way.

13. Inner Peace and Serenity:

14. Allow yourself to sink deeper into a state of inner peace and serenity. Release any worries or fears, knowing that you are supported and protected. Bask in the tranquil energy surrounding you and your baby, embracing this moment of connection and stillness.

15. Closing:

16. Return your focus to the here and now gradually. Flex your toes and fingers to extend your body in a gentle manner. After inhaling deeply a few more times, slowly open your eyes.

Conclusion:

Congratulations on completing your daily meditation practice! May this moment of tranquility and connection nourish you and your baby, filling your hearts with love and peace as you continue your journey through pregnancy. Remember to return to this practice whenever you need to center yourself and reconnect with the miracle of life growing within you.

∞∞§∞∞

12

Do's & Don'ts During Pregnancy

Do's During Pregnancy:

Finally, let's understand briefly what to do and what not to do.

1. **Eat a Balanced Diet:**

- Eat various foods, such as veggies, lean meats, dairy products, lean meats, whole grains, and natural goods.
- Please ensure you get enough folic acid, which is crucial for fetal development. It's found in leafy greens, citrus fruits, and fortified grains.

2. **Stay Hydrated:**

- Aim for eight-ounce glasses of water every day.
- Dehydration can lead to complications, so keep a water bottle handy and sip throughout the day.

3. Exercise Regularly:

- Take up low-impact activities such as swimming, walking, or stationary cycling.
- Prenatal yoga and modified strength training can help maintain fitness.

4. Get Enough Rest:

- Aim for 7-9 hours of sleep each night.
- Consider napping during the day if you're feeling fatigued.

5. Take Prenatal Vitamins:

- These supplements provide essential nutrients like folic acid, iron, and calcium.
- Your healthcare provider will recommend the proper prenatal vitamin for you.

6. Attend Regular Check-ups:

- Regular prenatal visits help monitor your health and the baby's development.
- Your healthcare professional should be contacted about any worries or questions you might have.

7. Educate Yourself:

- Read reputable books, attend childbirth and parenting classes, and seek advice from healthcare professionals.
- Recognize the changes your body will go through throughout

pregnancy and know what to anticipate from labor and delivery.

8. **Practice Stress Reduction:**

- Stress management methods include deep breathing, meditation, and prenatal massage.
- Think about the things that make you happy and calm.

Don'ts During Pregnancy:

1. **Avoid Smoking and Alcohol:**

- Smoking increases the risk of complications and congenital disabilities.
- Fetal alcohol spectrum disorders may result from alcohol use.

2. **Limit Caffeine Intake:**

- Excessive coffee intake has been associated with an increased risk of miscarriage.
- Limit caffeine from sources like coffee, tea, and sodas.

3. **Avoid Certain Foods:**

- Raw or undercooked seafood and eggs can harbor harmful bacteria.
- Unpasteurized dairy products may contain harmful pathogens.

4. **Be Cautious with Medications:**

- Some medications can harm the developing fetus.

- Always consult your healthcare provider before taking any medication, including over-the-counter drugs.

5. Avoid Hot Tubs and Saunas:

- Elevated body temperature can harm the developing baby.
- Saunas and hot tubs should be used cautiously and for short durations.

6. Be Careful with Cleaning Products:

- Choose cleaning products with mild or no chemicals.
- When using cleaning chemicals, make sure there is adequate ventilation and use gloves.

7. Watch Your Posture:

- I want you to please maintain good posture to prevent backaches and discomfort.
- Use supportive chairs and avoid standing or sitting for extended periods.

8. Avoid Heavy Lifting:

- Heavy lifting can strain your back and increase the risk of injury.

For specific advice depending on your health and pregnancy, always visit your healthcare practitioner. Every pregnancy is different, and every person's situation is diffferent.

∞∞∾∞∞

13

Daily Routine Chart

I have specially designed a chart to integrate into your everyday schedule easily. This well-organized manual sets tasks by your timetable to guarantee simplicity of use and optimal efficiency.

Morning Routine:

- **6:00 AM:** Wake Up
- **6:15 AM:** Morning Meditation (15 minutes)
- **6:30 AM:** Yoga Session (30 minutes)
- **7:00 AM:** Healthy Breakfast: Include whole grains, fruits, and protein-rich foods
- **8:00 AM:** Begin Work

Mid-Morning Break:

- **10:00 AM:** Stretching or Short Walk (10 minutes)

Lunch Break:

- **12:30 PM:** Nutritious Lunch: Balanced meal with vegetables, lean protein, and healthy fats
- **1:00 PM:** Relaxation Time: Listen to calming music or practice deep breathing (10 minutes)

Afternoon Break:

- **3:00 PM:** Snack Time: Fresh fruits, nuts, or yogurt
- **3:30 PM:** Gentle Stretching or Prenatal Yoga (15 minutes)

Evening Routine:

- **6:00 PM:** Light Dinner: Easy-to-digest meal with plenty of vegetables
- **7:00 PM:** Evening Walk or Prenatal Exercise Class (30 minutes)
- **8:00 PM:** Wind Down: Enjoy soothing music or a warm bath (15 minutes)
- **8:30 PM:** Relaxation and Mindfulness Meditation (15 minutes)
- **9:00 PM:** Bedtime

Hydration Tips:

- Drink plenty of water throughout the day, aim for at least 8-10 glasses.
- Consider adding herbal teas or infused water for variety.

Additional Tips:

- Take breaks as needed throughout the day to rest and recharge.
- Listen to your body and modify activities as necessary.
- Prioritize self-care and relaxation to reduce stress and promote

overall well-being.

Feel free to adjust the timings and activities based on individual preferences and schedules. This routine aims to promote physical and mental well-being while supporting a healthy pregnancy journey for working mothers.

∞∞∞∞∞

14

Resource

We extend our heartfelt thanks to the following sources for their invaluable contributions to this resource. Their expertise and dedication have greatly enriched the content, empowering and supporting expectant mothers on their journey through pregnancy and motherhood.

Coussons-Read, M. E. (2013). Effects of prenatal stress on pregnancy and human development: mechanisms and pathways. *Obstetric Medicine*, 6(2), 52–57. https://doi.org/10.1177/1753495x12473751

U.S. Department of Agriculture, U.S. Department of Health and Human Services, Vilsack, T. J., Sebelius, K., Van Horn, L., Fukagawa, N. K., Achterberg, C., Appel, L. J., Clemens, R. A., Nelson, M. E., Nickols-Richardson, S. (Shelly) M., Pearson, T. A., Pérez-Escamilla, R., Pi-Sunyer, F. X., Rimm, E. B., Slavin, J. L., Williams, C. L., Davis, C. A., McMurry, K. Y., . . . Sebelius, K. (2010). *Dietary guidelines for Americans.* https://health.gov/sites/default/files/2020-01/DietaryGuidelines2010.pdf

National Center for Biotechnology Information. (n.d.). https://www.ncbi.

nlm.nih.gov/

Square Roots. (2020, June 10). *Square Roots | Being Healthier Humans.* https://squareroots.com/

Sovren.Media: Premium video + social media. (n.d.). https://sovren.media /search/staypositive/

Shnuggle. (n.d.). *Shnuggle - Clever Baby products.* https://www.shnuggle .com/

Natural living for women - Natural-living-for-women.com. (2023, January 28). natural-living-for-women.com. https://natural-living-for-women. com/

Vocal. (n.d.). Vocal. https://vocal.media/

ConqueringMotherhood.com. (2023, September 12). *Helping new and expecting moms through pregnancy, babies.* Conquering Motherhood. https://conqueringmotherhood.com/

Quotesera - Quotes that will inspire you. (n.d.). Quotesera. https://quotes era.com/

Chiropractic Works. (n.d.). *Chiropractor | Watkinsville, GA & Athens, GA.* https://www.chiropracticworks.com/

Admin. (2024, February 8). *Reduce class size now – class size matters.* https://reduceclasssizenow.org/

Guru, M. (n.d.). *Mindfulness and meditation.* Mindfulness and Meditation. https://www.mindfulness-and-meditation.com/

Dmitri's Restaurant. (2022, October 12). *Dmitri's Restaurant | Come for the food, stay for the atmosphere.* Dmitri's Restaurant - Come for the Food, Stay for the Atmosphere. https://www.dmitrisrestaurant.com/

Home | Rays Reviews. (n.d.). Ray Reviews. https://www.rays-reviews.com/
   New World. (2024, February 8). New World. https://neovisnost.com/

Easiio. (n.d.). *Sflow.io | AI video makerblog to video, ppt tovide.* Sflow.io | AI Video MakerBlog to Video, Ppt Tovide. https://sflow.io/

15

About Author

Rose Rey is a passionate writer and devoted parent of two Loving Children, whose journey through the ups and downs of parenting has inspired her to share her experiences and insights. With 17 years of experience as a Senior Research Scientist in the pharmaceutical industry, Rose skillfully integrates evidence-based practices into her parenting advice, making it both relatable and effective. Her commitment to personal growth is reflected in her decade-long practice of meditation and Neuro-Linguistic Programming (NLP), which have enriched her communication skills and deepened her connections with others.

In her free time, Rose enjoys traveling and spending nights under the blinking stars, drawing inspiration from diverse cultures for her writing. Her love for writing stems from a desire to provide practical and helpful information to parents navigating the early years of their children's lives. In her book, Rose combines personal experiences, professional expertise, and extensive research to offer practical solutions and heartfelt advice to new parents. Her goal is to empower parents, helping them feel confident and informed as they embark on the incredible journey of motherhood.

16

Conclusion

As we bid farewell to the pages of this transformative journey, let's take a moment to bask in the profound wisdom and unwavering courage we've encountered along the way. From the first flutter of life within to the triumphant cry of new beginnings, each chapter has been a testament to the indomitable spirit of motherhood.

With every turn of the page, we delve deeper into the depths of our souls, uncovering stowed away saves of solidarity and strength we never knew existed. Through the hardships, the tears shed, and the victories celebrated, we've become more grounded, savvier, and profoundly associated with the beautiful excursion of bringing new life into this world.

As you close this book, may you carry the lessons learned, cherished memories, and the dreams nurtured within its pages. Let them serve as guiding stars on the horizon of your motherhood journey, illuminating the path ahead with hope, love, and unwavering faith.

Know that you are not alone on this journey. You are part of a vast sisterhood of mothers who have walked this path before you, whose love and support surround you like a warm embrace. Draw strength from their wisdom, find solace in their stories, and know that together, we are stronger than we could ever be apart.

So, as you embark on this next chapter of your journey, let your heart be filled with gratitude for the gift of motherhood, the privilege of shaping the future, and the boundless love that flows between you and your child. Embrace each moment with joy, wonder, and the knowledge that you are capable of miracles beyond your wildest dreams.

Dear Beloved Readers,

As we come to the end of this incredible journey together, I am filled with gratitude for the privilege of sharing these pages with you. Your presence, dedication, and commitment to growth have made this experience extraordinary.

As we part ways, I ask for your support in one final endeavor: sharing your thoughts and experiences by leaving a review for our book. Your feedback is invaluable to me and the countless other mothers who may embark on this journey in the future.

By sharing your audit, you are helping spread the news about the groundbreaking force of parenthood and offering direction and backing to the individuals who might require it most. Your words can inspire and engage others in their parenthood process.

Whether you found solace in the stories shared, discovered newfound strength within yourself, or felt a sense of connection and camaraderie, your review can make a difference. So please take a moment to share your thoughts, your insights, and your heartfelt reflections.

From the bottom of my heart, thank you for being a part of this incredible community. Your support means more than words can express, and I am deeply grateful for the opportunity to share this journey with you.

Hope we will meet again in the next chapter of Life.

With love and appreciation,

Rose Rey.